EMMA ROSE SPARROW

A Dusting of Snow

By Emma Rose Sparrow

Editor-in-Chief: Connor Chagnon
Sterling Elle Publishing
Bradford, Massachusetts
ISBN: 1500698067
ISBN-13: 978-1500698065

A DUSTING OF SNOW

An Emma Rose Sparrow Book

A DUSTING OF SNOW follows the story of a woman who reluctantly rises to face a wintery day. But she finds that things are a bit more interesting than she had planned.

A mysterious trail brings her on a personal journey that allows her to soak in the wonderful discoveries that a snowfall can offer.

If you are an adult bookworm who is looking for an interesting read or a book lover that enjoys a book that can be read over and over, this book is for you.

It is hoped that you find this book worthy of adding to your collection.

Enjoy your read!

EMMA ROSE SPARROW

TABLE OF CONTENTS

ACKNOWLEDGMENTS

Don't you just love the fact that a good book allows you to be transported to a new place, all while sitting in your favorite chair?

Books can bring us across to the other side of the world. Or they can show us things in our own backyards that we didn't take the time to notice.

For thousands of years, writers have worked to bring the joy of reading to those who appreciate a good story. Each year, hundreds of authors take their first try at writing and thousands of bookworms bring those books into their homes.

Great gratitude is given to all of the authors in the world. And a huge "thank you" is given to all of the book lovers around the globe.

If it were not for readers like you, the art of writing would be lost.

~Emma Rose Sparrow

CHAPTER 1: SEASONS

While I very well knew that it was morning and time to wake up, I kept my eyes closed. Curled up with my favorite comforter, the bed just felt too darn comfortable to leave at the moment.

Last night, I had heard a news report that the first snowfall may have been heading my way. I had mixed feeling about that.

I wasn't quite ready for snow because I love autumn. The explosion of colors on trees is nothing short of amazing. And I'm able to wear my favorite sweaters.

I also love springtime. It's lovely to see how the flowers begin to bud. I enjoy watching the trees wake up from their winter's hibernation. I like taking walks in the fresh, springtime air.

Just as much, I also enjoy summertime. Sunsets are simply marvelous. And what smells more invigorating than fresh cut grass?

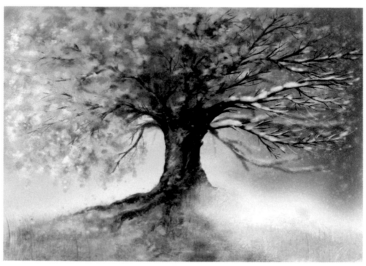

So, with a love of spring, summer and autumn, that bring us to talk about winter. I can sum it up in one word: "Eh".

Why do I think that winter is "Eh"? Well, to begin with, days are shorter. Add to that the fact that the sky is often gray. And I should mention that I'm not particularly fond of the cold.

So this morning, I stayed in bed thinking

about the prospect of facing the first snowfall.

I did eventually rise from bed. I also showered, dressed and ate a satisfying breakfast. It was only after the last piece of French toast sat in my stomach, that I decided to take a peek outside.

I stood at the door with my hand on the doorknob. I will confess that I was hesitating. If I looked and saw snow, that would mean at least 3 months of winter. Was I ready for that?

I slowly pulled the door open, with my eyes half closed. It wasn't overly gray. That was a good sign. My eyes lowered to look at the ground. There was a good dusting of snow.

It was only then that I remembered how beautiful winter can be.

The snow was perhaps an inch deep. Just

enough to create a nice, white blanket across the lawn. The canopy of trees held snow as well. It was pristine. And it was crisp and clear. I must admit that from my doorstep, it looked quite beautiful. So, perhaps I was wrong that winter was so bad.

It was time to venture out for a bit.

CHAPTER 2: FROSTING ON A CUPCAKE

It took me quite a while to get bundled up for the winter weather. After twenty minutes, there I stood, looking like the Pillsbury Dough Boy.

I had on 2 layers of slacks, 3 layers of shirts and 2 very thick socks on each foot. On top of that, I had on my snow boots and snow coat. And of course, I also had my gloves, hat and one very thick, woolen scarf.

The weather report on TV told me that the temperature would be slightly cold but not freezing.

I may have been a tad overdressed. I was sure that I'd be just fine if I were to be dropped off in the Artic. So, I'd be perfectly okay for a short walk into the yard.

I scanned the view from the front landing. What a sight! The world looks so splendidly different when it's blanketed with white fluff!

Every inch of ground that was green yesterday was now covered with crisp, clean snow. Taking in a deep breath, the air was cool and invigorating. There was a serene silence, as if the world had not quite woken up yet.

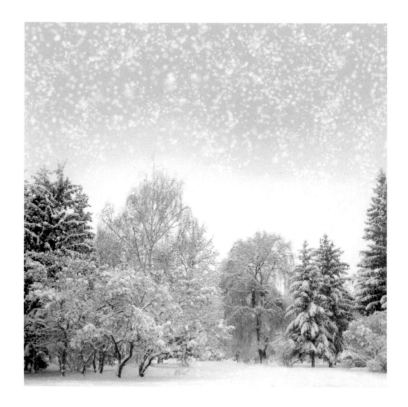

Tiny flakes began to drift downward. They fell so slowly, it was as if they were lazy and not sure if they truly wanted to land on the ground.

It's really quite amazing when Mother Nature powders the earth with a dusting of snow. It reminded me of a couple of things.

First, I thought about how a snowfall was like smothering frosting on a plain cupcake. This snow was like the perfect amount of vanilla icing on a chocolate dessert.

Another way to think about it, is that a blanket of snow is like an artist brushing thick, shiny white paint all over his canvas. It's like having a whole new landscape to begin anew.

I decided it was time that I have a closer look.

CHAPTER 3: THE TRAIL

The first thing to really catch my eye was a trail of tiny footprints. They ran straight through the yard and toward an area of trees.

I took care to stay to the side of the trail, as to not disturb it. Each step that I took caused a crackling noise as my boot would depress into the frosty snow.

I wondered if perhaps a young child had been outside playing in the snow. However, it was a bit too early in the morning for that. And if a child had been out here, he or she didn't build any snowmen. And the snow was unbroken except for the trail.

As I studied the tracks, I realized that they were not technically footprints.

I was looking at a paw prints. But I

couldn't be sure what type of animal had created them.

I decided that they could not have been made by an adult deer. The tracks were too small for a large, full grown animal.

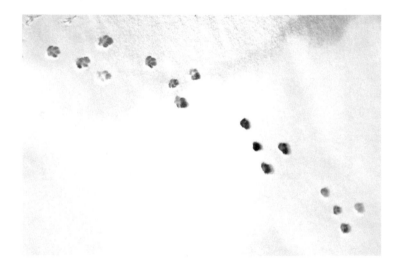

Maybe a fawn walked through the yard. But if so, why weren't there tracks of the mother deer?

I then considered the possibility that the tracks were made by a chipmunk or a squirrel. But something about it didn't seem to fit; I had never seen tracks like these before. This was quite a mystery.

I took a look back toward the house. I'd stay close. But I just had to find out where these tracks led to. I would follow them. Just a bit. Maybe I would find something.

CHAPTER 4: A FLASH OF RED

With such thick winter clothes on, I felt like I was waddling more than walking. But I persisted. My boots were holding up quite nicely. The many layers of my clothing, along with my snow coat, were keeping me warm.

I rewrapped my woolen scarf and adjusted my gloves. After taking a deep breath, I exhaled with a silent whistle. I was curious if I could see my breath.

A puff of steam rolled out of my mouth. That caused me to crack a smile. Satisfied that I was a human fog machine, I continued to follow the trail.

As I approached the tree line of a wooded area, a flash of red caught my eye. I knew what I had wished to spy, but I didn't want to get my hopes up.

Very slowly, I looked up toward the trees, to see if my guess was right. What do you know? Sometimes I do get it right!

There before me, was the most stunning cardinal bird.

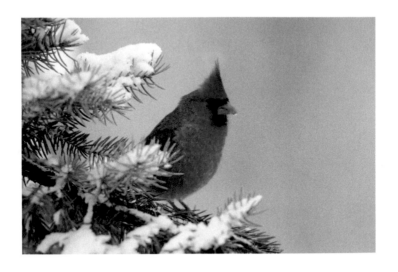

It sat perched on an Evergreen branch, composed and unmoving.

Its red was a shiny crimson. The black around its beak was deep and sharp. The crest on the top of its head stood up at attention. What a lovely sight!

This was a male. Females are not so flashy. They are a pale brown with just a touch of red on the wings.

Cardinals can often be seen in pairs. So I wondered where his lady friend was. Maybe she was off to collect food.

I had read that cardinals love to eat birdseed from feeders. If they can't find any seed, they will feast on insects, grain, fruit and even sap.

These birds are so beautiful and exquisite that 7 states in the U.S. have named the cardinal as their official state bird.

I stood in silence, waiting to see if he would sing. Researchers have identified 12 distinct cardinal songs that are repeated over and over among them.

A chirpy melody rang out over the stilled air. It sounded like, "Dooo, deet, deet, deet, deeeeeet."

He repeated it 3 times and then soared off. Maybe his female companion had found some seeds.

CHAPTER 5: SNOW ON THE BELLY

I stayed in place for a moment, staring at the branch where the cardinal had sat. It was bouncing a bit, as his weight had shifted off of it. Then, I remembered why I was out there. Those mysterious little tracks.

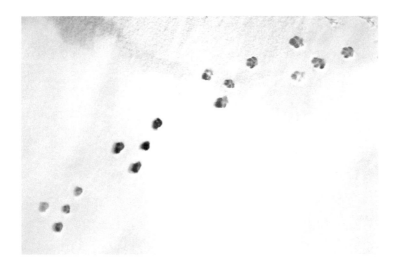

There they were, winding around the base of the tree and still heading off to somewhere. They were clear and easy to see in the fresh snowfall.

A very soft scattering noise got my attention. It was almost too faint to hear, but I did notice it. Whirling around, I thought that maybe I would see the critter that had made this trail. It turned out that I was wrong.

Running as if his life depended on it, I saw a small brown squirrel. This little creature was running swiftly through the snow. I imagined that he had dropped out of a tree, found the snow to be freezing and was racing for shelter.

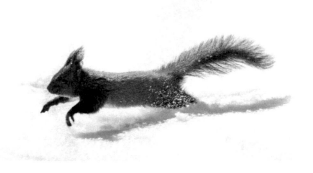

His little legs were so short; the small amount of snow must have felt like a blizzard to him. As he bounded along, he seemed to be trying to keep his belly off of the cold snow covering. I really didn't blame him; snow on the belly would be freezing!

Within just a breath of time, he had scurried up a birch tree.

There are over 1650 different species of squirrels and I couldn't possibly pretend to know them all. However I did think that this was a tree squirrel. They are given this name because they live in trees instead of in burrows like some other types.

The tree squirrel lives on every continent of the world, except for Antarctica.

He was a cute little guy and for his sake, I hoped that he was building a safe home in the high arching branches of the birch.

He would need the safety of the tree when we received the much heavier snowfalls of deep winter.

I took a moment to compare the squirrel's tracks to the tracks that I was following. They looked very different.   I felt confident that whichever type of small animal I was following was not a squirrel.

CHAPTER 6: PURPLE

I did realize that I couldn't follow the tracks in the snow forever. Just how far did this creature travel? Maybe food was scarce for her and she had to run a long ways to bring breakfast back to her babies?

I took a look back at the house. It was still in plain sight. That's good! The last thing that I wanted was to become lost in the snow. Or have people worried about me.

I inhaled a cleaning breath of fresh winter air and assessed how I was feeling. Not too bad! While I do tire out if I walk too much, I still had some energy in me and I'd go just a tad further.

A tiny pop of purple was visible in snow ahead. Purple? In the wintertime? I squinted my eyes to try and see it more clearly. No luck. I'd have to walk just a bit more to see what it was.

As I approached, a huge smile took over my face. I hadn't expected such a beautiful treat.

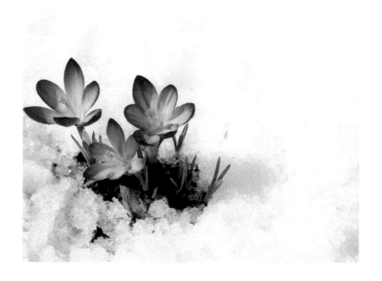

The most gorgeous sprig of crocuses were darting out of the light snowfall. Bright as anything, they shimmered like amethysts.

They stood up from the ground as if to say, "I defy this snowfall!"

I do remember hearing that some types of

crocuses bloom in the late autumn. That's what these must have been. And perhaps they were not aware that winter had come.

The word 'crocus' is Latin for saffron. While there are many types of crocus flowers, the saffron spice is derived from one of them: the saffron crocus flower.

Saffron is a rare and expensive spice that is used in recipes like seafood soups and rice dishes.

I took a moment to study the beauty of this amazing flower. The color contrasted so delightfully with the clean, white snow.

Just as I thought that maybe I would turn back and head home, I looked down at the tracks in the snow. They were saying, "You did it!"

CHAPTER 7: THE NOSE TWITCH

Right there, next to the crocus flowers, the tracks had stopped. I almost didn't believe that I had come to the end of the trail. Okay, then. It was time to find out who or what I had been following.

From what I could see, the small paw prints had stopped at a snow covered stack of thick scrub.

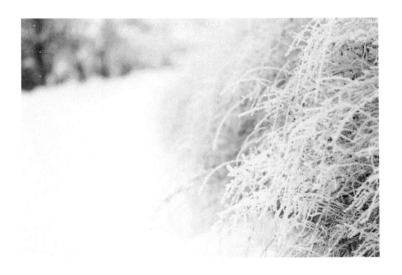

Tiny ice crystals had formed on the thin

branches, creating a tiny winter wonderland for whatever woodland animal decided to call this place home.

There was a gentle stirring of noise. Then, low and behold, a tiny nose popped out from the branches. Keeping very still, I watched as a pair of eyes appeared. The body soon followed.

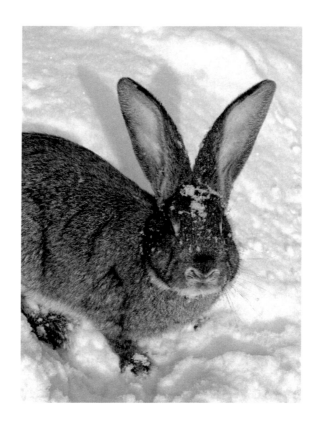

The most charming rabbit had stepped forward. She was sturdy and a bit plump. Her ears stood at attention. I couldn't help but smile at the scattering of snow that was atop her head.

She looked at me as if to say, "May I help you, my dear?"

Her eyes were very friendly and she stood patiently waiting for my answer. Not wanting to scare her off, I made sure to keep my voice low. With a whisper, I informed her, "I found you."

She wiggled her nose at me and casually stayed planted in place. Her expression was one of calm. As if it were no big deal at all that I had traversed the snow covered lawns to finally locate her.

I realized, of course, that she had no idea that I enjoyed my journey so much. She didn't know about the beauty that I had seen on my way to her. I wished that I could have told her about the red cardinal, the squirrel and the crocuses.

But instead, I softly thanked her for allowing me to enjoy the morning. It was fun to follow her little paw prints. I let her know that I appreciated the chance to notice the beauty in the wintertime.

Her nose twitched one more time, which I am certain meant "You're welcome" and she scurried back to her safe nesting area. With a huge smile and a stomach that was growling for a warm lunch, I headed back home.

ABOUT THE AUTHOR

Emma Rose Sparrow lives in a small New England coastal town with her two sons. She enjoys many creative ventures, including design and writing. She wishes to personally thank each and every one of her book readers for keeping the art of reading alive.

OTHER BOOKS IN THIS SERIES BY EMMA ROSE SPARROW

What the Wind Showed to Me

The Sandy Shoreline

Autumn's Display

Three Things

Down by the Meadow

Made in the USA
Monee, IL
05 September 2020

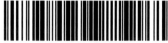